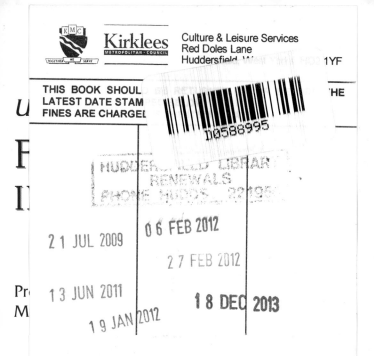
Published by Family Doctor Pub
in association with t

IMPORTANT NOTICE

This book is intended not as a substitute for personal medical advice but as a supplement to that advice for the patient who wishes to understand more about his/her condition.

Before taking any form of treatment YOU SHOULD ALWAYS CONSULT YOUR MEDICAL PRACTITIONER

In particular (without limit) you should note that advances in medical science occur rapidly and some of the information about drugs and treatment contained in this booklet may very soon be out of date.

Family Doctor Publications, PO Box 4664, Poole, Dorset BH15 1NN

Medical Editor: Dr Tony Smith
Consultant Editor: Maria Stasiak
Cover Artist: Dave Eastbury
Medical Artist: Philip Wilson
Design: MPG Design, Blandford Forum, Dorset
Printing: Reflex Litho, Thetford, Norfolk, using acid-free paper

ISBN: 1 898205 94 9

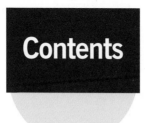

Contents

What is urinary incontinence?

Urinary incontinence is defined as bothersome urinary leakage causing a social or hygiene problem. It is a common condition which, although rarely life-threatening, is embarrassing and distressing, and may severely affect your quality of life.

Incontinence may be quite mild: the occasional leaking of small amounts of urine which does not cause embarrassment and which would therefore not be considered a problem. Or it can be very severe and may lead to people constantly having to wear pads to stay dry, avoiding normal activities such as sport or worrying about people noticing the smell of urine.

The causes of incontinence are very varied, and some are easily corrected – just as constipation can be easily cured with a better diet or a urinary infection with antibiotics.

Others may require surgery or long-term medication.

This book is written to help you learn about incontinence and how it may be treated. It is not designed to replace a consultation with your doctor but hopefully will help you understand the broader facts around the problem. It will also look at other urinary disorders such as recurrent cystitis or bladder pain, because not all women with bladder problems leak.

WHO IS AFFECTED?

Urinary incontinence is most commonly found in women who have had children but it can also affect children, men and women without children.

Urinary incontinence is estimated to affect around 2.5–3 million women in Britain. However, this figure is probably an underestimate, because there may be many women too embarrassed actually to admit that they have a problem. Some studies suggest that up to 30 per cent of women may be affected after pregnancy and childbirth.

SYMPTOMS

As well as leakage, there are a range of other symptoms of incontinence and bladder problems. You may have to pass urine more often than usual, which is known as frequency, and it may be painful or difficult to do so (dysuria). You may have a sudden and uncontrollable desire to pass urine. This is called urgency, and can lead to leakage if you don't reach a toilet in time. These are all common symptoms of cystitis, an inflammation of the bladder. You may have to get up in the night more often than normal to pass urine, which is known as nocturia, or you may have difficulties in emptying your bladder (voiding problems). You may have the sensation of wanting to pass urine but being unable to do so on demand, or you may suffer from hesitancy, which is a period of delay before you begin to pass urine.

WHY ARE PEOPLE SO RELUCTANT TO SEEK HELP?

Currently, the average time before a woman seeks medical help for incontinence is five years. She may be embarrassed by the problem, or may feel that it is 'to be expected' after having children, and may think that nothing could be done anyway. Or she may learn to 'manage' the problem, for example, by emptying her bladder frequently to prevent there being enough urine in it to leak.

But you should be reassured that there is a great deal of help available, from your GP, from specialist incontinence clinics and from local continence advisers who work in the community. Treatment options are very wide and range from simple changes in lifestyle to surgery. Some improvement in symptoms is possible for nearly everyone with incontinence. Help can also be given in managing the symptoms more effectively.

CASE HISTORY: SARAH

Sarah Hunt is a 36 year old who has had problems with leaking urine when she coughs. Her problems started after the birth of her second child when she was 30. At first she noticed slight leakage when she attended her aerobics class which meant that she had to stop doing step exercises. Over the next three years the problem increased, so she stopped going to the gym altogether. She eventually went to her GP for help after her problem became so bad that she leaked in public after picking her daughter up. When she saw her GP, she was having to wear sanitary towels whenever she went out, and her friends made a standing joke about her always using the toilet before going out.

Sarah was referred to her local hospital where she underwent urodynamics which showed her to have urodynamic stress incontinence. At this time Sarah was unsure about whether she wanted more children so she was referred to a physiotherapist who taught her pelvic floor exercises. After four months of these exercises, she is now able to control her problem. When she goes to the gym she wears a large vaginal tampon which stops her leaking during aerobics.

Case history: Dorothy

Dorothy Evans is a 65-year-old woman who went to see her GP because she was always going to the toilet. She was well known in most of the local shops as she often used their toilet when out shopping. She found that if she didn't void frequently she felt that she would leak and, on occasions, did leak before she found a toilet. Her GP sent her to a Continence Adviser for a supply of incontinence pads. However, her Continence Adviser recommended that she be assessed at her local hospital. The urodynamic tests showed that she had urodynamic detrusor overactivity.

Dorothy started taking an anticholinergic medication (a medication that blocks the action of the nerves on the bladder muscle) and bladder drill was commenced. She can now manage to shop without using the toilet. She no longer carries changes of underwear in case she leaks.

KEY POINTS

✓ Incontinence is a common problem

✓ It leads to a range of symptoms

✓ Women are often reluctant to seek help

✓ There is a great deal of help available

How the bladder works

It is important to understand how the bladder works, because there are many different types of incontinence, which may have quite different causes.

ANATOMY OF THE BLADDER

The bladder consists of a flexible sac of muscle (the detrusor muscle). Urine is produced in the kidneys and passes into the bladder through the ureters. The urine is then stored in the bladder until it is released. During storage the urine is retained in the bladder by a ring of muscles at the bottom of the bladder, called the urethral sphincter, which squeezes shut. The bladder neck, the area where the bladder and urethra meet, is partly supported in its position by the pelvic floor muscles which form a sling in the pelvis, helping to support the bladder, vagina and rectum.

The pelvic floor helps to hold the urethra in position on the underside of the pelvic bone. In this position, the raised pressure in the abdomen caused when you cough or sneeze is transmitted to the urethra, as well as the bladder, and has an equal effect. This is known as the pressure transmission theory and forms the basis of our understanding of continence. The pressure transmission theory is also the principle on which most surgical operations are based.

Bladder function is highly complex. It requires coordination from several parts of the brain and involves both involuntary and voluntary activity. This can be illustrated by looking in more detail at the urethral sphincter. This is made up of two parts each with a different function. The inner sphincter is made up of involuntary muscle; the brain operates this without conscious thought. It maintains a constant steady pressure, squeezing the urethra closed.

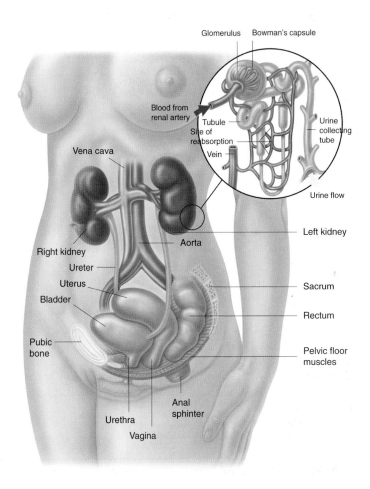

Normal female urinary anatomy and insert of kidney nephron. The kidneys filter waste products from the blood, which are excreted as urine.

It is helped by the lining of the urethra which is folded inwards many times so that when compressed it will give a watertight seal. The outer sphincter is made up of muscle which is under more voluntary control and it is this, along with the pelvic floor, that can be consciously squeezed when trying to prevent leakage. It is capable of very strong contractions but only for a short period of time. The muscle can be fatigued and this is why a sneezing fit may cause

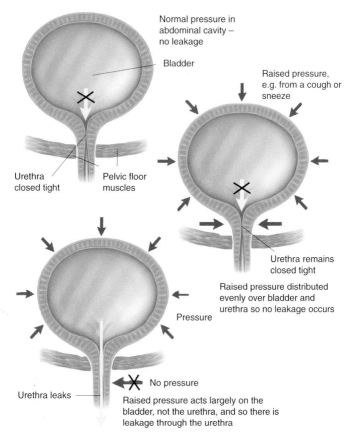

Normal pressure in abdominal cavity – no leakage

Bladder

Raised pressure, e.g. from a cough or sneeze

Urethra closed tight

Pelvic floor muscles

Urethra remains closed tight

Raised pressure distributed evenly over bladder and urethra so no leakage occurs

Pressure

No pressure

Urethra leaks

Raised pressure acts largely on the bladder, not the urethra, and so there is leakage through the urethra

Pressure transmission theory in abdominal/pelvic cavity.

leakage only after the third or fourth sneeze.

DEVELOPMENT OF BLADDER CONTROL

A newborn baby will empty his or her bladder about once an hour under reflex control, which means that the bladder empties automatically when it feels full. This only involves the bladder and the nerves running between the bladder and the spinal cord – at this stage the brain is not involved. The sensory nerves are stimulated by the filling of the bladder. These nerves in turn are connected to the motor nerves, which cause the bladder to contract. At the same time the urethra relaxes, allowing urine to pass from the bladder to the outside. The bladder fills and then empties; it is not yet used for storing urine.

As the baby gets older (around the age of two years), the brain develops and starts intercepting the messages from the sensory nerves. The brain can then suppress the impulse to make the bladder muscle contract and stop the reflex emptying of the bladder. The working bladder capacity will then increase and the bladder develops into a storage organ. Through potty training we learn what is acceptable behaviour and start to use the parts of our brain connected with bladder control.

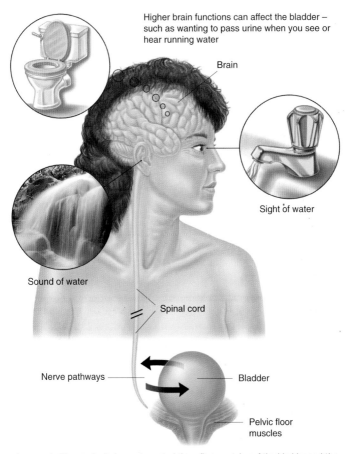

Higher brain functions can affect the bladder – such as wanting to pass urine when you see or hear running water

Brain

Sight of water

Sound of water

Spinal cord

Nerve pathways

Bladder

Pelvic floor muscles

As we get older, our brain learns to control the reflex emptying of the bladder and the bladder develops into a storage organ.

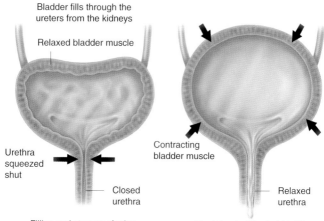

Bladder fills through the
ureters from the kidneys

Relaxed bladder muscle

Urethra
squeezed
shut

Contracting
bladder muscle

Closed
urethra

Relaxed
urethra

Filling and storage of urine

Emptying (voiding) of bladder

'Normal' bladder functioning.

Higher brain functions may also affect the bladder; for example, wanting to urinate when you hear running water.

WHAT IS 'NORMAL' BLADDER FUNCTIONING?

Bladder function can be thought of in two phases: filling and storage of urine, and emptying (voiding).

In filling, the urethra is squeezed shut while the bladder itself is relaxed, expanding as it fills with urine. In voiding, the urethra relaxes just before a contraction of the detrusor muscle in the bladder wall. The urine is then pushed through the urethra to the outside.

How often you pass urine is dependent on how much urine is produced as well as how much urine the bladder will hold. If you drink 1.5 litres a day and your bladder normally holds 400 millilitres (ml), then you will empty your bladder approximately four times that day. A bladder that holds only 100 ml results in passing urine fifteen times. If you drink twice as much, then you will need to empty your bladder twice as frequently. Normal frequency of voiding is up to seven times a day or not more than every two hours. In young women, the bladder normally holds 400–600 ml and is usually emptied when holding 250–400 ml. As people age, their bladder capacity tends to decrease, leading to increased frequency of micturition (voiding), especially at night.

HOW MAY PROBLEMS ARISE?

If the bladder neck and urethral sphincters are damaged (which may

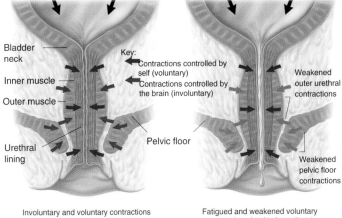

Involuntary and voluntary contractions
maintain continent bladder

Fatigued and weakened voluntary
contractions lead to incontinent
bladder

Urethral functioning and pelvic floor.

happen during childbirth), then they will not be as effective at sealing the urine inside the bladder. The bladder neck may also move downwards if the structures that support it are weakened and this will add to the problem; again this may result from childbirth, but straining may also be a cause (for example, with constipation or a chronic smoker's cough).

The bladder itself may be unstable or overactive (this is known as urodynamic detrusor overactivity). It is not known exactly what causes this, but it may be linked to loss of normal control of the bladder-emptying reflex, or nerve damage from childbirth or previous incontinence surgery. Anything that interferes with the parts of the brain involved in modifying bladder activity can affect bladder function; for example, a stroke or a spinal injury may interrupt the connection between the higher parts of the brain and the bottom of the spinal cord, resulting in a return to the reflex voiding pattern of a baby, incomplete emptying or loss of control.

Any kind of mass pressing on the bladder, for example, fibroids or a rectum full of faeces because of constipation, can cause problems.

These problems will all be looked at in more detail later.

KEY POINTS

✓ Normal bladder control is highly complex

✓ Bladder control is learned during early life

✓ How often you pass urine depends on how much you drink and the capacity of your bladder

✓ Continence relies on normal positioning of the bladder neck, normal nerve control of the bladder, and normal coordination and mental state (people who are unconscious or demented cannot control their bladders)

Why does urinary incontinence mostly affect women?

As we have seen, incontinence is a condition that can affect anyone. However, there are several reasons why women are particularly prone to it.

PREGNANCY

In pregnancy, the body's systems adapt to provide for the fetus as well as the mother. The bladder and pelvis undergo several changes during this time.

One of the first effects of pregnancy is to increase the amount of urine produced by the kidneys. This results very early on in an increase in the frequency of passing urine. Other hormonal effects lead to a general relaxation of the tissues in the pelvis, allowing the pelvis to become more flexible during the pregnancy and birth. The bladder may not empty as well during pregnancy as a result of the pressure effects. These changes may reduce the natural barriers to

bacteria which can lead to an increased occurrence of urinary tract infections.

As the uterus enlarges, increased pressure on the bladder leads to a need to pass urine more frequently. In about a third of women this increased pressure leads to leakage. This leakage usually stops with the birth of the baby, and is not linked with incontinence after childbirth.

Pregnancy can also lead to damage to the nerves controlling the muscles in the pelvis. In some women, the damage appears not to heal and this may be one of the causes of subsequent problems.

CHILDBIRTH AND BREAST-FEEDING

Childbirth itself can damage the muscles and supporting structures in the pelvis. During a vaginal delivery there is stretching of the side walls of the vagina and of the

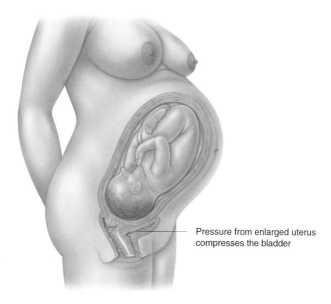

Pressure from enlarged uterus compresses the bladder

Pregnancy increases pressure on the bladder.

muscles of the pelvic floor. These muscles and tissues may not recover completely and this can cause loss of support for the uterus (womb) and the bladder neck which may eventually lead to prolapse of the uterus.

As the baby descends through the birth canal, damage may be caused to the pudendal nerve, which controls the muscles of the pelvic floor and runs around the edge of the birth canal, and this may lead to incontinence.

Breast-feeding helps to burn off the excess weight put on during pregnancy; it also helps pass on important nutrition and antibodies to the baby. Breast-feeding also delays the return of normal periods. This is sometimes relied on as a form of contraception, in that the chances of conceiving while breast-feeding are reduced as ovulation is less likely to occur. This delay in return to normal function of the ovary also means that the amount of oestrogen circulating is less. The reduction in circulating oestrogen may mean that it takes longer for the pelvis to recover from any damage as the tissues in the pelvis are oestrogen sensitive.

At the present time, there is no way to predict accurately which women are at risk of developing incontinence after childbirth. Various factors that may influence the effect of childbirth on your pelvis include the number of children that you have had, the type of delivery you had, how much the babies weighed, how long you were in labour and how long you pushed for. The first vaginal delivery carries the greatest risk, but even with this most women have no long-term symptoms. Instrumental deliveries (forceps and Ventouse) do carry a higher risk than normal deliveries. Caesarean section seems to spare some of these effects, but the benefit is lost after repeated pregnancies.

Something that does seem to be effective in minimising the risk of incontinence after childbirth is using pelvic floor exercises (see 'Finding out what's wrong' on page 15). These need to be taught properly and practised frequently. Most doctors feel that doing pelvic floor exercises before delivery may help to prevent symptoms. They need to be continued long term afterwards to be totally effective.

THE MENOPAUSE

At the menopause the ovaries cease to function and oestrogen levels in the blood fall dramatically. This can be responsible for the symptoms commonly associated with the menopause such as hot flushes and night sweats. It also has an effect on the pelvic tissues, which are oestrogen sensitive. As oestrogen levels drop, the muscles and tissues

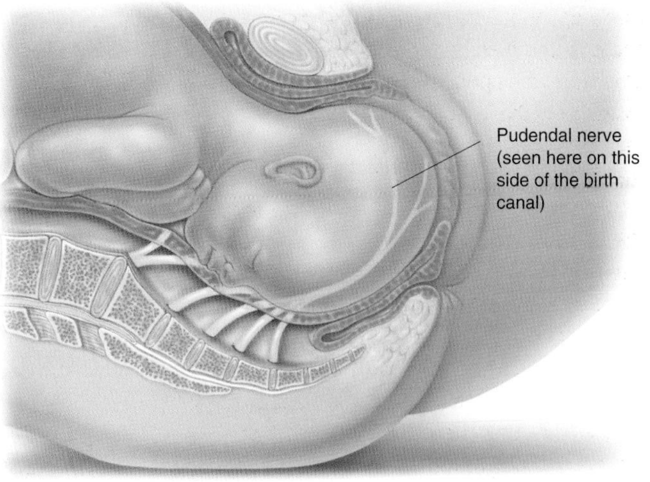

Pudendal nerve (seen here on this side of the birth canal)

Childbirth can cause damage to the pudendal nerve and this may lead to urinary incontinence.

in the pelvis thin and lose some of their previous strength. This particularly affects collagen, which is a supporting protein, in the skin. This results in loss of support for pelvic organs such as the bladder, bowel and womb, and may eventually cause vaginal prolapse.

Treatment with hormone replacement therapy may help to reverse these changes, but will not cure the problem, because once the collagen has weakened it will never totally go back to its former strength.

One other long-term effect of low oestrogen is atrophic vaginitis, which is a condition in which the vaginal walls become thin and inflamed. This results in itching and soreness. Atrophic vaginitis may be associated with changes in the bacteria within the vagina. The vaginal discomfort may lead to irritation around the urethra and so to increased frequency of passing urine.

INCREASED LIKELIHOOD OF INFECTIONS

The pelvic anatomy of women increases the likelihood of bladder infections, because the passage between the bladder and the outside, the urethra, is relatively short. This makes it easier for bacteria to enter the bladder. Sex may also help bacteria get into the bladder by pushing them upwards during intercourse.

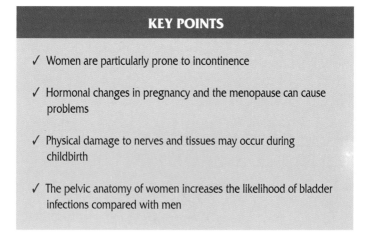

KEY POINTS

✓ Women are particularly prone to incontinence

✓ Hormonal changes in pregnancy and the menopause can cause problems

✓ Physical damage to nerves and tissues may occur during childbirth

✓ The pelvic anatomy of women increases the likelihood of bladder infections compared with men

Finding out what's wrong

WHERE TO GO FOR HELP

If you are suffering from incontinence, even only slightly, and it is affecting the way that you live, then you should ask for help. Your GP is the first port of call. He or she may be able to identify a cause such as a urinary infection and give you treatment. More often, you will be referred for specialist assessment at your local hospital or through the local District Continence Advisory Service. This service is responsible for treating most patients in the community. This is done through the running of community-based clinics and liaison with both GPs and hospital services. The continence advisers are a group of health-care workers who work specifically in

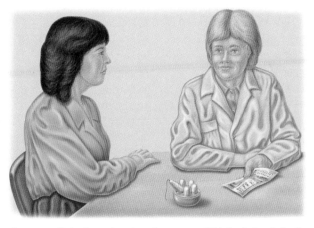

If you are suffering from urinary incontinence, your GP is the first port of call.

treating incontinence. They are trained nurses who have developed specialist skills in assessing and treating the condition. They are usually responsible for teaching and following up pelvic floor exercises, bladder drill and self-catheterisation.

Local continence advisers are also responsible for supplying aids and appliances (see page 60). This is done through liaison with the health authority supplying and the district nurses distributing the appropriate pads, pants or appliances.

INVESTIGATING THE PROBLEM

As we have seen, incontinence can have several different causes and, before treatment can begin, the doctor will need to find out exactly what is causing your particular problem.

One of the first things that will be checked for is a urinary tract infection, because this is easily treatable and can cause false results in later urodynamics tests.

The main aim of investigation is to find out if you have stress incontinence caused by weakness of the bladder neck, or urge incontinence caused by an unstable bladder. It may not be easy to tell from your symptoms alone, because these can be variable and one individual may have a mixture of both types of problem. If this is the

case, treatment may be started and then the tests repeated to see what progress is being made.

The tests will also pick up other rare forms of incontinence. Women with recurrent infections or with other bladder symptoms may also need investigating before proper treatment can be started.

Simple tests

A simple way to check the bladder function is to fill in a five-day chart that measures how much you drink and how much urine is passed, along with the frequency of urination. This is called a frequency volume diary and shows quickly and accurately how the bladder normally functions. The diary may in itself pick up the cause of the problem; for example, someone developing diabetes will show increased drinking and increased frequency of voiding. Inadequate fluid intake can also show up: this leads to highly concentrated urine, which irritates the bladder, producing symptoms of frequency and urgency. It can also predispose you to urinary tract infections, because passing only small quantities of urine diminishes the body's natural defences against bacteria entering the bladder.

Leakage can be measured with a pad test. A weighed sanitary towel is worn for about an hour with a full bladder. During this time you do a

KINGS COLLEGE HOSPITAL FREQUENCY VOLUME CHART

Time	Day 1 In	Out	W	Day 2 In	Out	W	Day 3 In	Out	W	Day 4 In	Out	W	Day 5 In	Out	W
6am															
7am				175	400		175	300			250		175	300	
8am	175	350		175			175			175					
9am															
10am						W							175		
11 am	160			175	250		160	200		160	150			150	
12 am	160		W												
1 pm	200	300		160			160	100		160	100		160	50	
2 pm				160	150					160					
3 pm								50			100				
4 pm	175			175	150		175			175	50		175	200	
5 pm			W												
6 pm	175	200		160			200	100		175			160	150	
7 pm					200		200	150			150				
8 pm								150		200					
9 pm	175	200		175						175			160		
10 pm					225		175		W		250			300	
11 pm		150						250			100				
12 pm															
1 am															
2 am															
3 am															
4 am								100							
5 am															

You may be asked to fill in a frequency/volume chart. This records your fluid intake, (In) urine output (Out) and leakage (W) during the day.

series of basic exercises such as sitting down and then standing up, walking up and down stairs, or washing the hands. The pad is then reweighed to calculate the weight and hence the volume of urine lost.

Urodynamics

The standard tests performed to assess bladder function are referred to as urodynamics. They measure the relationship between pressure and volume in the bladder and

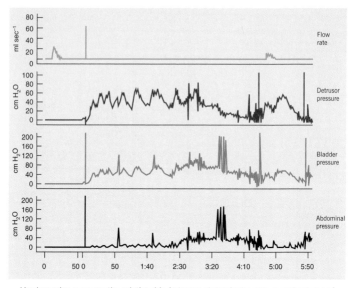

Urodynamics measure the relationship between abdominal pressure and volume of urine in the bladder.

whether or not these are normal.

When urodynamic tests are performed, you have to attend the clinic with a full bladder, and pass urine into a special toilet that measures the urinary flow rate. You are then examined and a small pressure (detector) transducer is placed in the bladder and one in the back passage. Although this is often embarrassing it should not be painful. The bladder is then filled through a catheter so that it is full again within five minutes. During this time the pressures from the two transducers are recorded. When the bladder is full again, simple tasks such as coughing or jumping are performed to see what happens to the pressures and whether there is leakage. Lastly the bladder is emptied into the special toilet with the pressure lines still in place for a 'pressure flow plot', which allows analysis of bladder pressure during urination.

Although nobody likes the thought of these tests, they can usually be performed relatively easily and with dignity. The doctors and nurses who perform them are all skilled in the techniques and try to make the tests as tolerable as they can.

In some hospitals, cystometry (measurement of the pressure and volume of the bladder when full and during emptying) may be used with

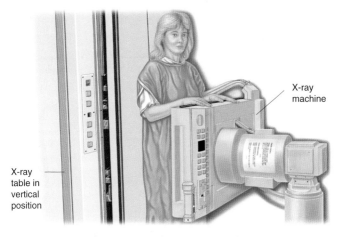

Patient having an X-ray of the pelvic region.

X-ray machine

X-ray table in vertical position

X-ray imaging to look at the relationship of the bladder neck to the leakage during coughing. This test is of particular value with women who have had previous surgery or complicated problems, and is known as video urodynamics.

The information provided by urodynamics is limited, because it only provides a snapshot of the bladder's function over a relatively short period of time (approximately twenty minutes while the test is performed). Ambulatory urodynamics allow the conditions that provoke problems to be mimicked under test conditions. It normally takes four hours and allows the bladder to fill with urine naturally, rather than a fast 'retrograde fill' through a catheter. It is currently available only in a few hospitals in the UK.

Imaging techniques

There are two procedures that are commonly used to find out whether other parts of the urinary tract have been affected. These tests look for damage caused by infections or from the passage of urine the wrong way up the ureter from the bladder to the kidney, and they also check for kidney stones.

The first is called an intravenous urogram. This involves injecting dye into a vein in the arm, which is then excreted through the kidneys. A series of X-rays (radiographs) are taken at timed intervals. The dye outlines the kidneys, ureters and bladder, allowing the anatomy of the whole area to be observed. The second technique is an ultrasound scan which is used to look at the bladder and the kidneys (see page 20).

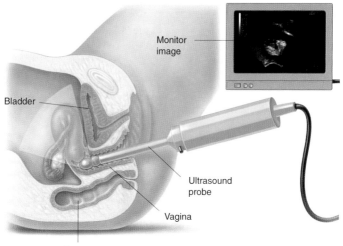

Ultrasound scan.

Cystoscopy

A cystoscopy is performed to look at the inside of the bladder. A cystoscope is a narrow telescope which is passed into the bladder through the urethra.

There are two types: a flexible cystoscope under local anaesthetic or a rigid cystoscope under a general anaesthetic. The advantage

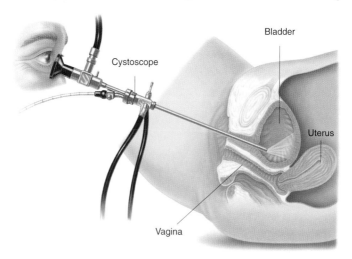

Cystoscopic examination of the bladder.

of the rigid cystoscope is that it allows samples of the lining of the bladder to be taken for analysis (see page 20).

Nerve tests

Very occasionally a test is performed to assess the nerve supply to the muscles of the bladder neck. This test, electromyography, involves the insertion of a needle electrode into the muscle of the urethra to measure electrical activity in the muscle.

KEY POINTS

✓ Investigation is necessary to distinguish between urodynamic stress incontinence, urodynamic detrusor overactivity and other causes of incontinence

✓ A frequency volume chart (urinary diary) is a simple way of showing how the bladder normally functions

✓ Urodynamics are standard tests carried out to assess bladder function

✓ Cystometry studies the pressure–volume relationship in the bladder

Stress incontinence

The most common type of incontinence is stress incontinence, which accounts for around 40–50 per cent of women with the condition. Leakage occurs with exertion such as coughing, sneezing or playing sports.

The most severe sufferers will leak with the slightest pressure on the bladder. Other women have a problem only during periods of extra exertion such as when playing sport. Fear of leaking will often stop women doing everyday activities such as aerobics or playing with grandchildren, and can be very restrictive.

A common way of women 'managing' the condition is to empty their bladders regularly so that there is never enough urine there to cause a serious problem. They are then able to avoid embarrassing wet patches by the use of pads so that a small leakage does not disrupt their lifestyle. But they may then find themselves having to visit every toilet between the shops and home, or working in an office where frequent trips to the toilet become embarrassing. Others seek help because they are no longer able to cope with the frequent changing of underwear or the prohibitive cost of buying pads.

WHAT CAUSES IT?

Stress incontinence commonly occurs as a result of a combination of weakening of the urethral sphincter or bladder neck, which seals the bladder between voidings, and a change in the position of the bladder neck. There may thus be a wide variety of causes: hormonal changes during pregnancy and the menopause, physical damage from childbirth, straining, as with a chronic cough or constipation. Many women have a mixture of stress incontinence and urge incontinence.

Normal | Stressed

Rise in abdominal pressure, e.g. cough or sneeze

The bladder neck is well supported and the muscle sphincter squeezed tight shut. A rise in abdominal pressure acts evenly on squeezing the bladder and sealing the urethra; there is no leakage of urine

The bladder neck has fallen and the muscle sphincter is strained, so a rise in abdominal pressure acts more by squeezing the bladder than sealing the urethra; urine then escapes

Stress incontinence occurs as a result of a combination of a weakening of the muscle sphincter seal and a change in the position of the bladder neck.

As we saw earlier (page 4), the urine inside the bladder exerts a pressure on the bladder neck, which squeezes shut to resist the pressure and retain the urine inside the bladder. In order to stay dry, the sphincters in the bladder neck must remain tightly closed when the pressure on the bladder from the outside increases from coughing, sneezing or laughing. Normally, the position of the bladder neck is such that any rise in pressure from coughing affects both bladder and urethra equally. If the bladder neck moves down from its normal position, the urethra is no longer compressed by the rise in pressure. This results in the sphincter mechanism being put under more strain and urine escapes.

Teenage girls are prone to an embarrassing but self-limiting condition called giggle incontinence, where they leak on laughing, but not at any other time. This condition is not properly understood, but it does not usually cause major problems and women can be reassured that it will resolve spontaneously without medical intervention.

TREATMENT

There are a wide range of treatments for stress incontinence, from physiotherapy to drug treatment to surgery. To decide which is best, doctors will look at when the problem occurs, what is causing it, and your needs and desires. For example, you may wish to reduce the leakage so that it can be managed with little disruption to your life, but may not want to embark on surgery, even though it could leave you completely dry.

Non-surgical treatments

• **Physiotherapy**: Physiotherapy should be available to all women. The type of physiotherapy commonly employed for incontinence is called pelvic floor exercise or training. This incorporates a series of exercises contracting the pelvic floor muscles, using repetition and endurance exercises designed to re-educate and strengthen the muscles in the pelvic floor, leading to increased support of the bladder and urethra. It is safe and effective with no side effects. It does,

NON-SURGICAL TREATMENTS

- Pelvic floor exercises (physiotherapy)
- Vaginal cones
- Biofeedback
- Electrical therapy
- Drug therapy

however, rely heavily on your motivation, and also needs proper teaching and follow-up. It is ideal for women awaiting, or unwilling to undergo, an operation or those medically unfit for surgery. Results of physiotherapy are not immediate and frequent regular exercises must be continued for at least 3–6 months to allow improvement, but maximum benefit is only achieved

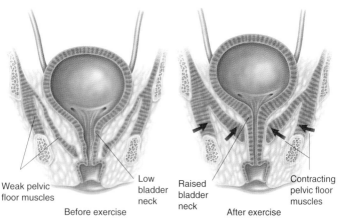

Weak pelvic floor muscles | Low bladder neck

Before exercise

Raised bladder neck | Contracting pelvic floor muscles

After exercise

Pelvic floor exercises re-educate and strengthen the muscles in the pelvic floor, and so increase support for the bladder and urethra.

by correct long-term usage.

Pelvic floor exercises should be taught by properly trained physiotherapists and continence advisers. You can be referred by your GP or you can see a physiotherapist privately without necessarily having seen a doctor. Normally you make several visits to the instructor to check that the contractions are being performed correctly and to help you to maintain motivation. The assessment usually involves an internal examination where your ability to squeeze is manually graded by the instructor, who will look at the strength of the contraction, the length of maximum contraction and the number of repetitions performed. Alternatively, a device called a perineometer may be used. This consists of a vaginal probe attached to a pressure gauge from which the strength of the contraction can be read off. Some women are unable to contract their pelvic floor muscles to command or are unaware of what the sensation of a contraction is, and these women require extra help with learning the skill.

Success rates vary but with good tuition and motivation up to 70 per cent of the women may be improved to their satisfaction, although only 25 per cent are completely cured.

• **Cones**: Weighted vaginal cones can also be used to strengthen the pelvic floor muscles, and may be particularly helpful in learning to identify the muscles of the pelvic floor. The cone is held in the vagina; when this can be done for two successive periods of 15 minutes,

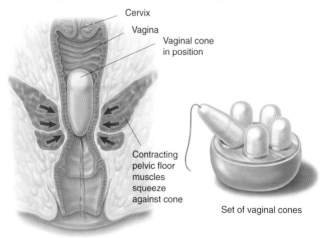

Cervix

Vagina

Vaginal cone in position

Contracting pelvic floor muscles squeeze against cone

Set of vaginal cones

Weighted vaginal cones can be used to strengthen the pelvic floor muscles.

an identically sized but heavier cone is substituted. There are from three to five different weights in a set of cones. Cones are usually easier to learn how to use than traditional pelvic floor exercises, and require less follow-up supervision. However, pelvic floor exercises still form an essential part of treatment. Although cones can be purchased through medical supply companies it is usually better to buy them through a continence adviser or physiotherapist. This is because not all women are suitable for cones and proper assessment is required first. If you have a large prolapse, for example, the cone can sit behind it without ever strengthening the pelvic floor muscles and in this case the cones are not beneficial.

- **Biofeedback**: Biofeedback may also help women to become more aware of their pelvic floor muscles. The use of a perineometer, as described above, is an example of biofeedback: seeing the reading on the pressure gauge change will help the woman to recognise what a contraction of the pelvic floor feels like, and will help her to learn to control the muscles.

- **Electrical stimulation**: There are currently three forms of electrical treatment: interferential, Faradism and maximal electrical stimulation (MES). The difference between the types of stimulation allows slightly different applications of the treatment, the choice of which should be left to the instructor. Interferential is normally only used in hospital and works by applying current through four electrodes, producing a cross-firing current. It can also be used for urgency or mixed incontinence. Faradism and MES use one or two electrodes and have the advantage that they can be used at home after initial supervision. These techniques provide 'passive' muscle stimulation to increase muscle tone, and allow women to become aware of the pelvic floor. They can be used under supervision or at home after the technique has been learned. The stimulation makes the pelvic floor muscles contract and, by feeling this happen, you will become more aware of where these muscles are and what they do.

- **Drug therapy**: In the past drug therapy has been thought to be unhelpful where the stress incontinence is caused by weakness of the bladder neck. However, where there is evidence of oestrogen deficiency, oestrogen hormone treatment may be an important factor in increasing the success of other forms of treatment such as pelvic floor exercises. It works by improving the strength of tissues in the bladder neck, vagina and pelvis, which weaken as a result of low oestrogen levels. However, it is not in itself a cure for incontinence.

Very occasionally a medication called phenylpropanolamine (which is contained in some common cold remedies) is used. It artificially helps the muscle in the bladder neck contract to maintain a tight seal. Like oestrogen, it is used in conjunction with other therapies to make up a whole programme of treatment for the individual. The use of this medication is, however, restricted because pelvic floor exercises achieve better results and have no side effects. A new drug is being developed that is similar to the antidepressant Prozac. Within the next year or two, it should be available to help people with minor but troublesome stress incontinence.

Surgical treatment

To date over 250 different operations have been described for treating incontinence. A number of factors are taken into account when deciding which is the best choice for a particular woman, including whether it is a first operation or repeat surgery, the facilities locally and the wishes of the patient. All surgery carries risks and, the larger the operation, the greater the risk of complications.

There may thus be a trade-off where a smaller procedure may be preferred because it is easier and quicker, even though the success

---

TYPE OF SURGICAL TREATMENT

- Bladder neck injections
- Vaginal repairs with buttressing
- Bladder neck suspensions
- Colposuspensions
- Sling procedures

---

rate may be lower. Smaller procedures also have quicker recovery times.

Incontinence operations divide broadly into five different classes of operation. Some operations require the surgeon to open up the abdominal cavity; in others the operation can be done through the vagina.

Abdominal procedures have higher success rates than the other types of operation, but also tend to take longer to recover from. They are considered bigger operations as they require an incision on the abdominal wall along the bikini line.

• **Sling procedures**: These operations pass a sling under the urethra and stitch it to the abdominal wall. There is a wide variety of materials used for the sling, from autografts (strips of material removed from another part of the body such as the rectus sheath) or artificial materials such as Teflon or Goretex tape. This is also an abdominal procedure.

Over the last eight years a new

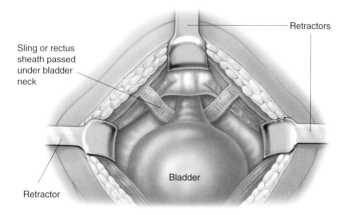

Sling or rectus sheath passed under bladder neck

Retractors

Retractor

Bladder

Sling procedure.

type of sling called tension-free vaginal tape (TVT) has been used. The advantages of the TVT are that the operation is much quicker and much smaller, and therefore the recovery is much quicker.

The results from the TVT suggest that this is as successful as conventional surgery, although long-term results are not yet available. There are also several other companies offering tape procedures that mimic the TVT coming on to the market.

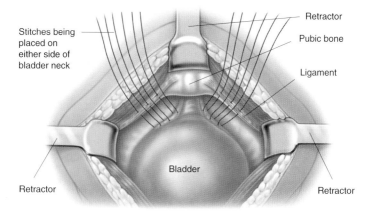

Stitches being placed on either side of bladder neck

Retractor

Pubic bone

Ligament

Retractor

Bladder

Retractor

Colposuspension.

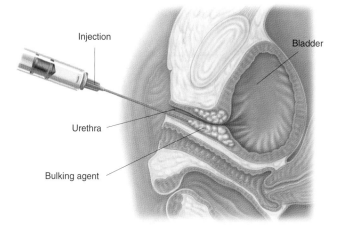

A bladder neck injection involves injecting a bulking agent into the area around the bladder neck, to provide support and increase pressure on the urethra.

• **Colposuspension**: Colposuspension literally means 'supporting the vagina'. This is achieved by carefully dissecting the bladder neck free of its attachments and passing stitches through the supporting structures at the side. These stitches are then tied to the ligament or to the bone itself on the inside of the pelvis. The operation takes place through an abdominal incision along the bikini line, and hence takes longer to recover from than the procedures above.

• **Bladder neck injections**: The simplest type of procedure is the bladder neck injection. This involves injecting one of a number of bulking agents around the bladder neck. The most commonly used substances are GAX bovine collagen (Contigen) or tiny silicone particles (Macroplastique). Some surgeons undertake this as a daycase procedure under local or regional anaesthetic, but more commonly it is performed under general anaesthetic.

This type of operation is aimed at increasing the resistance at the bladder neck by bringing the edges together so that urine cannot easily leak out. This type of operation has a relatively low absolute cure rate, although more often than not it does lead to some improvement. It is relatively easy to repeat if necessary and does not usually cause significant scarring.

Very occasionally, afterwards women have problems emptying their bladders, but this is usually transient and most women tolerate

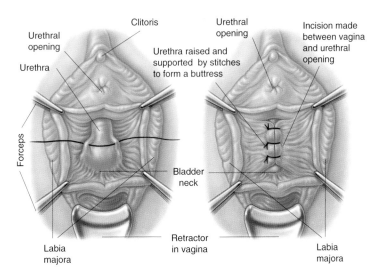

Clitoris

Urethral opening

Urethra

Forceps

Labia majora

Urethral opening

Urethra raised and supported by stitches to form a buttress

Bladder neck

Retractor in vagina

Incision made between vagina and urethral opening

Labia majora

A vaginal repair operation aims to reposition the bladder and urethra by pushing them up from below.

the injection well with little discomfort.

● **Vaginal repair**: The aim of a vaginal repair is to reposition the

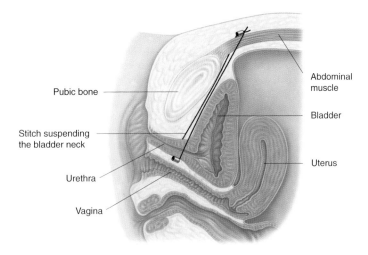

Pubic bone

Stitch suspending the bladder neck

Urethra

Vagina

Abdominal muscle

Bladder

Uterus

A bladder neck suspension aims to raise the level of the bladder neck.

bladder and urethra by pushing them up from below. This type of operation can be performed to repair a prolapse (where part of the vagina or the uterus has moved down into the pelvis) or to elevate the bladder neck to restore continence: restoring the bladder to its proper position.

Vaginal repair is a simple procedure to perform and patients recover rapidly. It is often initially successful and is currently the second most common type of operation performed. However, recent studies have cast doubts on its long-term success rate.

• **Bladder neck suspensions**: These operations aim to lift the bladder neck by passing two sutures on each side of the bladder neck and securing them above the muscle in the abdominal wall. It is a relatively straightforward procedure which is easy to perform and has low complication rates.

After bladder neck suspensions some women occasionally have problems passing urine. This depends on how far the bladder neck has been lifted, and is because the operation may partially obstruct the bladder neck, although this is not a permanent problem.

• **After surgery**: One of the most common side effects of this sort of surgery is transient obstruction, where the woman has problems emptying her bladder. In the short term this may happen to as many as 20 per cent of women. For most, however, it is no more than a minor set-back and, given a longer period of time, bladder function returns to normal. Simple retraining in how to empty your bladder properly may be needed, such as sitting with your legs further apart and tilting the pelvis by leaning forwards.

However, some women require a longer period of catheterisation (see page 46) to rest the bladder (usually around 10 to 14 days). Occasionally women need to be taught how to catheterise themselves if the voiding difficulties persist. This can usually be achieved easily and should be no more troublesome than having to change a tampon.

Most women agree that the inconvenience of having to catheterise is far less than the stigma and loss of self-esteem of the incontinence. Sometimes it is possible to predict who is at risk of voiding difficulties before surgery. In these cases self-catheterisation may be taught before surgery. (See page 46 for more details about catheterisation.)

The other complication of these operations is the development of irritative symptoms such as frequency and urgency. This occurs in around 10 per cent of women. Nobody understands the reason for this and it is not usually predictable. It is likely that, if you had frequency and urgency before the operation, then you will have it afterwards, or it may get worse.

Using devices to contain leakage

Another approach to the management of stress incontinence focuses not on curing the problem but on containing it by physically limiting leakage. Over recent years, there have been several attempts to market devices that have not been commercially successful. These devices may come back on to the market in the future. Many are disposable, and may eventually be

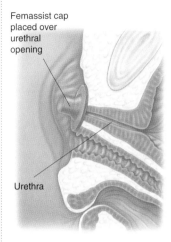

Femassist cap placed over urethral opening

Urethra

Femassist device.

available over the counter.

One type of device acts as a physical barrier to the urethra. The Reliance acts as a plug. It is held in place by a small balloon at the bladder neck and sits in the urethra in a similar fashion to a catheter. This initially needs to be sized by an experienced medical practitioner or nurse to ensure it fits. These devices are disposable and are thrown away after being removed for voiding.

Another example of this type of device is the Femassist, which is a cap that sits on the outside of the urethral opening, and is held in place by suction. This device is reusable and only needs simple hygiene measures such as washing to keep it clean.

Another type of device (Introl) is designed to elevate either side of the bladder neck. Again the correct

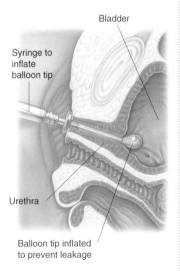

Bladder

Syringe to inflate balloon tip

Urethra

Balloon tip inflated to prevent leakage

Reliance device.

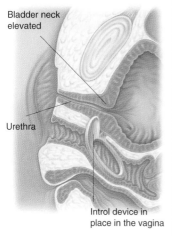

Bladder neck elevated

Urethra

Introl device in place in the vagina

Introl device.

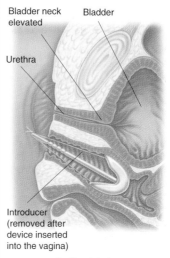

Bladder neck elevated

Bladder

Urethra

Introducer (removed after device inserted into the vagina)

Contigard device.

sizing and fitting requires an experienced operator. This device comes in several different sizes that allow the ring to sit comfortably inside the vagina. An Introl has two prongs that press up either side of the bladder neck of variable lengths to allow the correct elevation.

A vaginal sponge can also be used. This is known as a *contrelle*. This acts like a large tampon and helps press the urethra up against the pubic bone to stop leaking. It is a similar device to the Contigard, which also elevates the bladder neck.

The advantages of these devices is that they are simple to use and allow the woman total control; they only need to be used when required. Sometimes women find that using an ordinary tampon may compress the urethra enough to allow continence.

The use of a tampon may be applicable when doing aerobics or during times of physical exertion. It is important to remember that the manufacturers do not recommend the use of tampons at times other than periods, and that they need to be removed after use to reduce risks of infection.

KEY POINTS

✓ Stress incontinence accounts for 40–50 per cent of women with incontinence problems

✓ It can be caused by anything that weakens the bladder neck support – usually as a result of childbirth – causing its position to drop

✓ Pelvic floor exercises can help up to 75 per cent of women

✓ There is a range of surgical operations to treat the condition

✓ Devices are available to contain leakage

Urge incontinence

The second most common type of incontinence is urge incontinence. Urgency is the sudden and uncontrollable desire to pass urine; if a toilet is not reached in time there may be leakage. This is the 'I want to go . . . oops I've leaked' situation. Occasional urgency is normal and it is only a problem if you feel that the symptoms are affecting your lifestyle or you have recurrent infections.

In most cases, urge incontinence results from an instability of the muscle in the bladder wall (the detrusor muscle). The condition is known as urodynamic detrusor overactivity. The detrusor muscle contracts to force urine out through the bladder neck when you pass urine. Normally it does not contract until there is an appropriate time for passing urine. But if it is unstable or overactive, it may contract involuntarily, resulting in the sensation of urgency and the need to void more often than normal

(frequency). Incontinence can result from urodynamic detrusor overactivity if the bladder neck is weak or is opened by the force of the contraction. The problem tends to wax and wane, often being worse during the winter months.

The involuntary contractions can be triggered off by a variety of things. Coughing is one of them, and thus a person with urodynamic detrusor overactivity can go to their doctor with the symptoms of stress incontinence (because they leak when they cough). Things such as the sight and sound of running water can also be a trigger. The fuller the bladder, the more likely it is that involuntary contractions will occur.

The two major types of urgency are urodynamic detrusor overactivity (motor urgency) with involuntary contractions and sensory urgency, in which the bladder feels very uncomfortable but there is no actual leaking. The

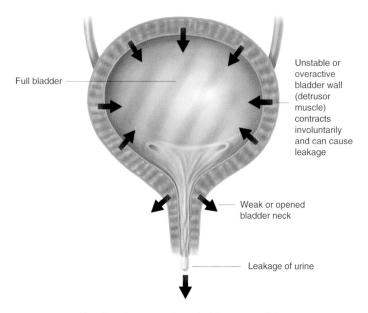

Urge incontinence – urodynamic detrusor overactivity.

differentiation of these two types of problem requires a variety of tests called urodynamics (see page 17), although there are other features to suggest what the problem may be.

What causes it?

In most cases we do not know. Urodynamic detrusor overactivity may be related to loss of normal control of the bladder-emptying reflex or relative overactivity of one of the nerves supplying the bladder. Nerve damage and neurological conditions such as a stroke or multiple sclerosis can cause the bladder to contract in an unstable way. If there is a known neuro-logical cause for the instability, the condition is known as detrusor hyperreflexia.

Often people who develop the condition have a history of bed-wetting as a child or have always had a 'weak bladder'. This may be a result of poorly learned bladder training as a child. Quite often other members of the family have had problems as well.

Women who have had previous incontinence surgery may also be prone to the condition. The original surgery may have partially blocked the bladder neck to stop leakage. The bladder's response is to cause the muscle to thicken, and in some cases the normal control mechanism is lost, resulting in an unstable bladder.

TREATMENT OPTIONS

Treatment of urodynamic detrusor overactivity is based on trying to stop the bladder contracting. This may be achieved by behavioural therapy or by the use of medication. Both of these approaches tackle the symptoms rather than the cause of the problem and neither offers a cure.

Behavioural therapy

Behavioural therapy works by re-educating the brain to control the bladder more effectively, in particular by suppressing the involuntary contractions which cause urge incontinence.

The mainstay of behavioural therapy is bladder drill. First the bladder is emptied. A target time is then set, usually an hour, during which the woman is then not allowed to use the toilet (even if this means leaking). After the hour has passed the woman must pass urine. This is then repeated so that a pattern of regular toileting is established. The time is slowly increased as each target is repeatedly met. The aim is to achieve three-hourly voiding.

Bladder drill has been shown to be highly effective in treating urge incontinence when taught as an in-patient in hospital, with up to 85 per cent of women being dramatically improved. It does, however, require a very high level of motivation and commitment, along with encouragement from staff. Consequently, on leaving hospital there is a very high relapse rate as women return to their normal lifestyle, which does not always allow for a strict toilet regimen. There is usually less encouragement and support outside a hospital, although bladder drill is also taught and supervised in the community by physiotherapists, continence advisers and nurses. Despite the problems with maintaining progress, bladder drill remains an important tool in the management of an unstable bladder.

Biofeedback can be used to help with bladder drill. Electrical sensors can be used to detect bladder activity, which will help the patient to learn what the sensation of the bladder contraction is, so that they can more easily learn to suppress it.

The same principle of bladder drill can be applied to bedwetting. In this case it involves knowing when the bedwetting occurs and setting an alarm clock for beforehand. When incontinence is regularly avoided the time can be gradually increased.

Drug treatment

The most common type of medication used for the treatment of an unstable bladder is the anti-cholinergic drugs. These preparations act by blocking the impulses between the nerves controlling the bladder and the bladder muscle. In this way the response of the muscle to stimulation is damped down, and the drugs act almost like a shock absorber. As this treats the symptoms rather than the cause of the problem, treatment may need to be long term or even for life.

The major problems with anticholinergic medications are side effects, because they can affect other parts of the body. The most common side effects are a dry mouth, blurred vision, constipation, heartburn, palpitations and, if the drugs act too successfully, difficulty in passing urine. They can't be used if you have closed-angle glaucoma, and some people find that the tablets make them drowsy or tired. Even so, although most people get some side effects (and to some extent these must be anticipated if the medication is to be successful) the benefits make it worth while.

If side effects are a real problem, a tricyclic antidepressant (amitriptyline or imipramine) may be tried instead. These medications also have anticholinergic effects but the side effects are not so severe. Newer anticholinergic medications, such as tolterodine, propiverine and trospium chloride, have become available recently and may have fewer side effects.

Many of these anticholinergic medications are now available in slow release form and therefore as once daily dosing, which acts further to reduce the side effects. Not every medication suits every individual and therefore the medications may need to be tried to find out which is the best for any individual.

Another approach to managing the condition is by using an artificial hormone called desmopressin. This hormone signals to the kidneys to slow down their urine production, which thus reduces the rate of bladder filling. This is particularly helpful for the night-time as urine production should be naturally reduced, allowing sleep through the night.

The problem with this type of treatment is that it cannot be used continuously; if the kidneys produce

SIDE EFFECTS OF ANTICHOLINERGICS

- Blurred vision
- Dry mouth
- Constipation
- Urinary retention
- Heartburn
- Palpitations

less at night they must compensate and produce more during the day. Desmopressin is therefore used predominantly in children who wet the bed or in adults whose symptoms are worst at night. It is not usually given to people who may be at risk if they retain extra fluid, e.g. people with high blood pressure or heart problems.

Oestrogens may also be used in postmenopausal women as part of a management strategy.

Changes in diet and lifestyle

Smoking is known to irritate the bladder and make an unstable bladder worse. Caffeine and alcohol have a doubly bad effect, because not only do they stimulate the bladder, but they also stimulate the kidneys to produce more urine. Thus the instability of the bladder is increased, and it also has to cope with a bigger workload. Caffeine is found not only in coffee but also in tea and some fizzy drinks, and these can worsen symptoms.

A possible compromise as regards alcohol is to switch from beer or other long drinks to spirits or wine, so that at least the volume of liquid passing through the bladder is reduced.

For some people, simple adjustments to their living arrangements may be sufficient. For example, a woman of reduced mobility may leak in the morning because her bladder is full and she cannot walk to the bathroom without significant effort. Supplying a commode by the bed may solve the problem.

Surgery

The simplest form of surgery would be to insert a suprapubic catheter (a catheter passed through the wall of the abdomen rather than through the urethra), which allows the bladder to be kept empty but reduces the risk of infections from the catheter. Very occasionally an operation called an augmentation (or clam) cystoplasty is performed. This is a last resort, as it can be complicated and there is a high risk of on-going problems. The operation involves stitching a patch of bowel into the bladder which can then act as a shock absorber for the bladder contractions.

KEY POINTS

✓ Urge incontinence results from an instability of the muscle in the bladder wall

✓ In most cases the cause is unknown

✓ Treatment may be with behavioural therapy or medication

✓ These treatments tackle symptoms but do not offer a cure

✓ Changes in diet and lifestyle may help

Problems with emptying the bladder

Broadly speaking, problems with emptying the bladder (or 'voiding') can be divided into two groups. If the bladder muscle is weak or does not contract as it should, then the bladder will not empty properly. Or if the bladder neck cannot relax or is scarred, it will be difficult for the bladder muscle to force urine past it. In both cases the bladder may not empty completely. These processes can occur separately or together.

SYMPTOMS

Recurrent cystitis

A common complaint which indicates a difficulty in emptying the bladder in women is recurrent cystitis, because the problem reduces the normal protective mechanisms against bladder infection. Bacteria are normally washed away from the bladder and the area outside the urethra during voiding. If the bladder is not emptying properly, the bacteria will stay there for longer and be more likely to cause infection.

Hesitancy

This is the symptom of wanting to void and the delay between trying to start voiding. In an extreme form it leads to strangury which is pain associated with trying to void. This is more commonly associated with prostatism, a male disorder.

SYMPTOMS OF VOIDING DIFFICULTIES

- Recurrent infections
- Hesitancy
- Urgency and frequency
- Overflow (dribble) incontinence
- Bladder pain

Urgency and frequency

If the bladder does not empty properly it reduces the available space, which may then result in increased frequency of micturition and in nocturia (getting up at night more than normal to pass urine).

Urgency may also be a problem (see Glossary on page 65).

Retention

Retention is a condition where the bladder cannot empty. If this occurs as a sudden event then it is usually very painful and requires immediate action to prevent damage to the bladder as a result of prolonged over-filling.

Chronic retention can also occur, which is usually relatively painless. Retention occurs because the bladder outlet becomes obstructed, for example, as the result of a fibroid pressing on the urethra, or the bladder is unable to create enough muscle power to enable emptying.

The first part of treatment is to drain the bladder using a catheter. Once that is done, the doctor may then arrange tests to determine the cause, for example, a mass pressing on the bladder. In this case, the tests include a blood test to check that the kidneys have not been damaged by the pressure exerted on them by the bladder, and an ultrasound scan. Urodynamics (see page 17) may also be used.

Overflow (dribble) incontinence

When the bladder is unable to empty, the pressure inside it will eventually build up so much that urine leaks 'off the top'. This is known as overflow incontinence and is non-acute retention. There may be an almost continuous leakage of urine (dribble incontinence).

This sort of problem is mostly seen in men with prostate problems but can occur in women, particularly if there is pressure on the bladder from a large uterine fibroid. Overflow incontinence can also occur in association with other medical problems such as multiple sclerosis where the bladder coordination is lost. In these cases, the bladder contracts to empty but at the same time the urethral sphincter contracts to stop the bladder emptying (see pages 8–9).

Dribble incontinence may also be caused by fistulae (see page 57).

Bladder pain

Bladder pain caused by voiding difficulties is normally an intense desire to empty the bladder, which is called urgency. The pain is normally 'suprapubic' which is just above the pelvic bone. Infections are often associated with this intense urgency; classically, however, infections also cause a burning pain during passing of urine. In severe cases there may even be a dull ache left after voiding.

CAUSES OF VOIDING DIFFICULTIES

Drugs

Medications such as antidepressants can suppress the bladder's ability to contract. If the bladder function is normally relatively weak, this can tip the balance between being able to empty or going into retention.

Nerve damage

Damage to the nerves supplying the bladder can alter the bladder muscle's ability to contract; hence a chronic or severe back problem (e.g. a slipped disc) can trigger off difficulties.

CAUSES OF URINARY RETENTION AND VOIDING DIFFICULTIES

- Drugs
- Nerve injury/neurological problems
- Childbirth
- Epidural anaesthetic
- Fibroids/pelvic masses
- Constipation
- Surgery
- Narrowing of the urethra
- Prolapse
- Weak detrusor muscle
- Urinary tract infections

Childbirth

Urinary retention can commonly result from childbirth, particularly after an epidural anaesthetic, which will decrease bladder nerve function. Women who have had an epidural should have an indwelling catheter to protect the bladder until normal sensation returns (about 12 hours).

There is also an increased risk after a forceps delivery, or when there is marked trauma to the perineum and vagina which may make passing urine painful and hence the woman avoids voiding and eventually becomes unable to do so.

Fibroids/pelvic masses/constipation

Fibroids are a common gynaecological condition that occasionally causes difficulties in emptying the bladder. Fibroids are benign tumours growing in the womb. If the fibroids cause an external obstruction to the bladder neck, it becomes increasingly difficult to empty the bladder. As the fibroids grow, the problem increases until the woman goes into retention. Any other lump or mass in the pelvis (constipation, for example) can cause similar problems.

Surgery

One of the most common causes of temporary voiding difficulties is pelvic surgery, and continence surgery in particular. When the bladder neck is lifted to reposition it, there is always an element of obstruction. If the pressure of the contraction of the bladder muscle cannot overcome this, then there will be difficulties in emptying the bladder. Most women who have had a colposuspension, for example, will notice that they void at a slower rate after surgery.

Postoperative voiding difficulties can be divided into short-term or long-term problems. Around 20 per cent of women have some minor degree of voiding dysfunction which will settle with careful catheter management. Of these around one per cent have long-term problems which require long-term treatment. The most successful way to manage the problem is self-catheterisation, which allows the woman to control her symptoms and gives her freedom to lead a normal life (see page 46).

Strictures to the urethra

Stricture or narrowing of the urethra is now relatively uncommon in women. It can occur if trauma or an infection damages the lining of the urethra which then heals leaving scarring. Strictures cause voiding difficulties by reducing the size of the urethra and thereby creating outflow obstruction. Urethral strictures will require an operation either to dilate or to cut the narrowing, but need to be carefully assessed before treatment to check that there are no other problems and to ensure that treatment will not damage the urethra further. Strictures often recur and sometimes require repeated treatment.

Prolapse

Prolapse can cause problems with bladder emptying by kinking and therefore obstructing the urethra; this is just like kinking a garden hose to stop water flowing out of the end. Correction of the prolapse then restores the bladder neck to its normal position to allow normal voiding. Often prolapse and incontinence coexist because the damage that causes prolapse also leads to stress incontinence.

Weak detrusor muscle

The detrusor muscle gets weaker with age and contracts less efficiently. The bladder wall also becomes stiffer. As a result the bladder functions less well. These are normal effects of ageing and are the reason that it takes longer for elderly people to empty their bladder as well as needing the toilet slightly more often.

Occasionally, the nerves to the bladder stop working properly, which stops the detrusor muscle from contracting properly. Nerve damage to the bladder occurs after urinary retention or as a result of nerve damage from diabetes, multiple sclerosis or a stroke. This may in itself not always lead to a problem because part of voiding is relaxation of the pelvic floor, which may be enough in its own right to allow emptying. Usually, however, women require active force to empty their bladders.

INVESTIGATIONS

Voiding difficulties require thorough investigation with urodynamics (see page 17). If there is the symptom of loin pain or there have been serious kidney infections, then tests will be performed to check that urine does not flow the wrong way up the ureter (from the bladder to the kidneys). Additionally, a test to check on the pressure in the urethra may be performed. This is called a urethral pressure profile.

If there is any doubt or there is a history of infections then a cystoscopy may be performed. This allows a doctor to inspect the inside of the bladder through a telescope, which is usually done under a general anaesthetic, and also allows small biopsy samples to be taken from the bladder for analysis.

TREATMENT

Often mild degrees of difficulty can be managed with simple advice. When sitting on the toilet make sure your legs are apart rather than having your knees together. Leaning forwards or even standing slightly may alter the angle of the bladder neck enough to allow better emptying. Waiting for two minutes after the initial void and then trying again may help. This is known as the double void technique.

More severe symptoms may require actual treatment. There are three approaches to the treatment of voiding difficulties:

1. Try to increase the force of the bladder contractions. This can be achieved in some cases using bethanechol, which stimulates the nerve fibres controlling the contraction of the bladder muscle. This may be effective if there are no signs of obstruction at the bladder neck or urethra.
2. Try to reduce outflow obstruction. This method would be used if there was a specific site of obstruction in the urethra such as a stricture, or narrowing demonstrated during investigation as mentioned above.
3. Third, and probably most commonly, catheters are used. They can either be used occasionally, or can remain in place long term.

Occasional self-catheterisation when properly taught in a healthy individual with normal dexterity is

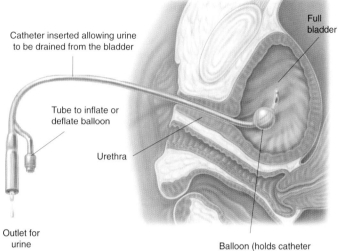

Catheter inserted allowing urine to be drained from the bladder

Full bladder

Tube to inflate or deflate balloon

Urethra

Outlet for urine

Balloon (holds catheter in place)

Catheterisation.

the best option. It gives you freedom to control your bladder symptoms with no more inconvenience than having to change a tampon.

THE USE OF CATHETERS

A catheter is a soft, flexible tube, thinner than a pencil, with a rounded end. When passed up the urethra into the bladder, it allows all the urine to flow out without any muscular effort.

Although initially the thought of having to catheterise is upsetting to most women, when they have learnt the technique and are confident, they find it far easier than expected. The technique requires a basic understanding of pelvic anatomy and being taught how to identify the urethra. Initially a mirror is helpful for this, but with time most women manage without. With practice inserting a catheter through the urethra is not normally painful.

The number of times you need to catheterise is dependent on how your bladder functions.

KEY POINTS

✓ Difficulties emptying the bladder may cause a variety of symptoms

✓ They can be caused by drugs, nerve damage, childbirth, fibroids or pelvic surgery

✓ Simple advice may be sufficient to deal with mild cases

✓ Self-catheterisation may be an effective way of managing the problem

Urinary infections

The urinary tract is made up of the kidneys, ureters, bladder and urethra; infection of any of these organs may spread to the others.

The symptoms of urinary tract infections may differ widely. Some women have no symptoms at all, and the infection remains hidden until it causes kidney failure. Other women are crippled with pain and 'cystitis', and may pass blood in their urine. Women experiencing more than three infections per year are defined as having recurrent infections.

What causes infections?

Bacteria are small organisms which are found everywhere. Normally they do not cause an infection when they are in their normal habitat. If the balance of bacteria changes then this may allow an overgrowth of one type and, in these circum-stances, it can cause damage that shows as an infection. It is not unusual to find bacteria in a normal woman's bladder. Cystitis is an inflammation of the bladder and can be the result of infection. The female urethra (the passage between the bladder and the outside) is relatively short, which allows easy access to bacteria found around the vagina and perineum (the area between the vagina and the anus). Quite often these are the same as the bacteria found in the bowel. When the bladder empties it washes them out of the bladder, and as the urine leaves the body it cleans the area just outside the urethra.

If the bladder does not empty fully these bacteria stay in the bladder and can start to multiply or colonise the bladder. If the bacteria increase in number they can then start to damage the lining of the bladder, producing inflammation.

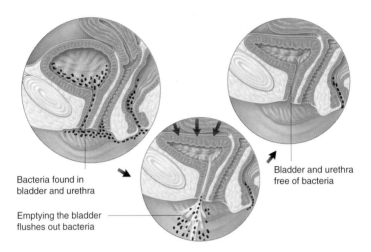

Bacteria found in
bladder and urethra

Emptying the bladder
flushes out bacteria

Bladder and urethra
free of bacteria

Emptying the bladder completely may help to wash out harmful bacteria.

This, in turn, causes the symptoms of burning and frequency characteristic of cystitis.

Thus difficulties in emptying the bladder are a major cause of infections. Another factor in infection is sexual intercourse. During intercourse, the bacteria normally present outside the urethra can be pushed into it and so spread up into the bladder. This is called auto- or self-infection. New types of bacteria can also be introduced from the man. Sex can also cause small abrasions which can give the bacteria a stronger foothold from which to colonise the bladder.

There are simple measures that can be used to avoid infections associated with sexual intercourse.

Emptying the bladder completely soon after sex may help to wash out the bacteria in the bladder. In order to gain the full protective effect, however, the bladder must be at least comfortably full. Just emptying a small drop out of the bladder will not wash all the bacteria away. You should also consider the type of contraception you use. Urinary infections can occur as a result of using the diaphragm and spermicide in around 10 per cent of women, and in some cases using condoms stops infections occurring. Some women are allergic to the most common spermicide, nonoxinol '9'. Non-allergic condoms can be used in these cases.

Simple hygienic measures may also help lessen the growth of

bacteria on the outside of the vagina, for example, always wiping from the vagina towards the anus after using the toilet. Douching is unwise, because it will normally remove the natural, helpful bacteria, allowing more harmful bowel bacteria to colonise, and may actually increase the risk of infection. The vagina is a self-cleaning organ and does not require detergents or perfumes.

Kidney stones are another rare cause of infections. If bacteria infect a stone then it is almost impossible to clear the infection. In these cases the stone needs to be removed. Infections are also more common in pregnancy (see page 11).

INVESTIGATION

When you see your doctor he or she will first confirm that you have an infection rather than some other condition such as interstitial cystitis (see below). To do this a urine sample will be sent off for testing before you are treated with antibiotics. The urine sample needs to be a mid-stream specimen. This is collected by starting to empty your bladder into a toilet and, when the stream is established, you catch a sample in a sterile container. The reason for discarding the first part of the stream is that this can be contaminated by bacteria on the skin and in the urethra. The mid-stream sample should give a representative specimen from inside the bladder. The results from the sample will be used to ensure that the correct antibiotic is being used.

If you get recurrent infections, repeated samples will be taken to build up a picture of the types of infection you get. This will suggest whether you are developing different infections, or whether the problem is the same infection that is not being adequately treated.

Women with proven recurrent infections require further investigation to exclude other causes of infection, such as chronic kidney infection. A frequency volume chart (see Urodynamics, page 17) may give important information on your bladder behaviour.

Urodynamics is routinely used to check, along with a cystoscopy, inside the bladder.

TREATMENT

In mild cases the infection will settle on its own, just requiring the treatment described below for the symptoms. Many women say that drinking a lot of water clears infections. It is more likely that it reduces the symptoms by keeping the urine dilute while the bladder is sore, allowing the body's natural defences to clear the infection. Bicarbonate of soda, barley water and cranberry juice are also commonly suggested as cures for cystitis: they may help to reduce the acidity of urine which may make it less painful to void.

Established infections will need adequate treatment with an appropriate antibiotic. Often doctors will treat empirically, which means they prescribe an antibiotic likely to treat the infection. This is because they wish to treat immediately rather than wait three days for confirmation of the type of infection and the correct antibiotic. Remember that because an antibiotic does not work on one occasion does not mean that it will not work in subsequent infections.

Having excluded any underlying cause for the recurrent infections there are two treatment options. First, low-dose antibiotics can be used at night in an attempt to keep the bladder sterile and treat any infection before it gets a hold. The second approach is to treat only when necessary.

If symptoms occur only after intercourse then an antibiotic can be taken either before or immediately afterwards. Alternatively, most women who have recurrent cystitis know when symptoms are going to develop up to 12 hours beforehand. In these cases taking a single dose of an antibiotic often cures the symptoms. If they persist then further antibiotics can be taken. Symptoms lasting longer than 24 hours normally mean that the infection is resistant to the antibiotic.

Very occasionally the infections are caused by bacteria such as *Ureaplasma* or *Mycoplasma*. These infections are not usually checked for and, if symptoms persist, a special sample of urine should be sent to the laboratory to look for them specifically. They may require long-term treatment with antibiotics for around three months.

INTERSTITIAL CYSTITIS

Interstitial cystitis is a relatively rarely diagnosed inflammatory condition of the bladder, the cause of which is far from clear. It causes bladder pain and mimics cystitis caused by an infection. It often causes frequency and urgency and can cause the bladder lining to bleed, leading to blood in the urine. Diagnosis is based upon several symptoms and signs, including changes to the bladder's capacity and increased bladder sensitivity, plus a biopsy or sample of the bladder wall, which will show an increase in inflammatory cells, particularly mast cells (a type of immune cell).

Interstitial cystitis occurs almost exclusively in women, raising the question of whether there is a hormonal influence. Most women with the condition (up to 95 per cent) are white, and symptoms start after the age of 20. This is around the age when many women become sexually active, which makes it more difficult to distinguish from recurrent infections.

Even though the cause of interstitial cystitis is unknown, the effects are now beginning to be understood. The bladder wall becomes inflamed and thickened. This may be as a direct result of an infection or because the body's defence mechanism acts against the cells of the bladder. It is these two ideas that have led to most approaches to treatment.

Treatment

Common treatments include long-term antibiotic treatment (for at least three months). This is to keep the bladder free of any infection while giving the bladder wall a chance to heal and recover. Alternatively, bladder antiseptics taken by mouth can be used to try to create an environment for healing.

Drugs known to reduce inflammation can be used and simple medications such as aspirin or aspirin-like medications may help. A greater anti-inflammatory effect is achieved using steroids such as prednisolone.

Another anti-inflammatory treatment involves using antihistamines, better known as a treatment for hay fever and stomach ulcers. The mast cells in the bladder wall release histamine, which is involved in producing inflammation. Antihistamines reduce the effects of this and consequently may improve symptoms.

There are many other medications such as antidepressants, anticholinergics and calcium antagonists that have been suggested for interstitial cystitis, as well as some operations. Unfortunately, the causes that trigger interstitial cystitis have not been identified and therefore medication can currently only treat the symptoms.

There are some lifestyle changes that appear to help. These are based on trying to identify trigger factors for the condition, such as caffeine. Avoidance of these substances can often be as effective as medication.

KEY POINTS

✓ Recurrent urinary tract infections are often related to sex or difficulties in emptying the bladder

✓ Simple hygiene measures can help

✓ Treatment is with antibiotics

✓ Recurrent infections may be confused with interstitial cystitis or vice versa

✓ Interstitial cystitis is a rare type of cystitis

Other problems associated with urinary incontinence

When a doctor sees a patient with incontinence for the first time, he or she will ask about other aspects of the patient's health as well, because some other conditions have a link with incontinence.

PERIODS AND FIBROIDS

You will be asked about your periods, because if these are heavy and painful it is possible that you may have fibroids. Fibroids are benign tumours growing in the wall of the womb. They are very

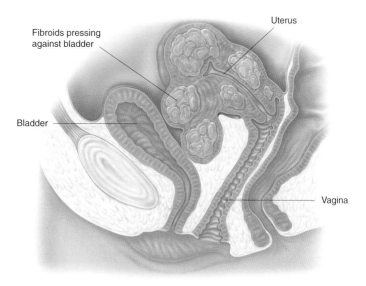

Fibroids can grow in the wall of the womb, displacing the bladder and increasing abdominal pressure.

common and usually do not cause problems. If, however, they do cause distortion of the pelvic organs then they can interfere with the bladder or your periods. In particular they can increase abdominal pressure and add to the displacement of the bladder neck associated with incontinence. If you are likely to need surgery for incontinence, this may be a good time to assess whether the fibroids also need treatment.

PROLAPSE

Prolapse is the movement of the vaginal wall from its normal position along with the bladder, bowel or womb. It is caused by damage to the ligaments in the

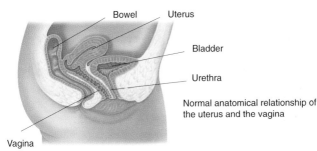

Bowel   Uterus

Bladder

Urethra

Normal anatomical relationship of the uterus and the vagina

Vagina

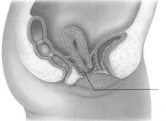

Uterine prolapse – the uterus sinks down through the vagina

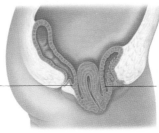

Cystocele – the front wall of the vagina falls and the bladder follows behind

Rectocele – the back wall of the vagina falls, bringing part of the bowel down with it

Prolapse is the falling or dropping of any organ from its normal position within the vagina.

pelvis. These ligaments act as guy ropes supporting the womb and the strength-giving layers overlying the bowel and bladder. The main causes of prolapse are childbearing and any condition leading to chronic straining (constipation, smoker's cough or being overweight).

There are several different types of prolapse and these are graded according to severity. A cystocele is a prolapse of the front wall of the vagina with the bladder following behind. Uterine prolapse refers to the womb coming down through the vagina. A rectocele is a prolapse of the back wall of the vagina with the bowel coming down behind.

Prolapse may occur on its own or in conjunction with other symptoms such as incontinence or difficulty passing a bowel motion. Common complaints include the feeling of 'something coming down' and discomfort or pain during sex.

Treatment of prolapse is dependent on several factors, including your wishes and how much the prolapse interferes with your life. The best results are usually obtained by surgery which aims to fix the organs back into their proper positions, but this is not always the most appropriate treatment. You may not have completed your family (and another childbirth could cause the prolapse to recur), may be unfit to have surgery, or may just not want it. Sometimes silicone

rings called pessaries can be placed in the vagina. If these cure symptoms they can be used on their own, just requiring changing every six months. A major drawback is that the pessary sits in the vagina and therefore sexual intercourse can be difficult.

DIABETES

Diabetes may affect the bladder in many ways, from causing frequency as a result of excessive drinking, to damaging the nerve supply to the bladder. In the latter case diabetes can cause urodynamic detrusor overactivity or difficulties emptying the bladder or both, depending on the exact effect of the diabetes on the nerves.

It is therefore important that, if you have symptoms of diabetes (thirst, frequency and weight loss), or if you have a strong family history of diabetes, you are checked for this.

IRRITABLE BOWEL SYNDROME

It is not uncommon to find that women who have bladder symptoms, particularly of an unstable bladder, also have bowel symptoms. Irritable bowel syndrome can cause a variety of effects from abdominal bloating and constipation to diarrhoea. The symptoms may vary from time to time and be related to other factors, such as stress or your periods. The first choice treatment for irritable bowel syndrome is to increase dietary fibre to encourage normal bowel action. Medications such as peppermint preparations and anti-spasmodics can be used to try to regulate bowel spasms. Laxatives may be used if constipation is a problem.

Drug treatment for an unstable bladder may worsen constipation (see page 38) and this must be borne in mind if it is likely to be a problem.

BACK PROBLEMS

Lower back problems can cause pinching of the nerves supplying the bladder as they exit the spinal canal.

This in turn can alter the functioning of these nerves, and may lead to difficulties in emptying the bladder. Hence a back problem may present as a urinary problem. Treatment of the bad back by properly supervised physiotherapy can reduce the pressure caused by entrapment of the nerves and lead to an improvement in symptoms.

FISTULAE

A fistula is an abnormal track between two cavities, e.g. the bladder and vagina, and can lead to incontinence. This can allow urine to leak directly into the vagina rather than being stored in the bladder.

Fistulae occur for several reasons. In developed countries the most common cause of fistulae is as a result of cancer or radiotherapy for

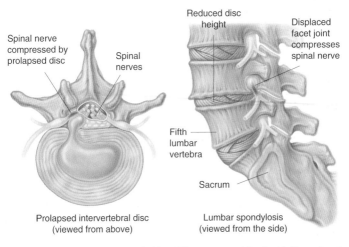

Spinal nerve compressed by prolapsed disc

Spinal nerves

Reduced disc height

Displaced facet joint compresses spinal nerve

Fifth lumbar vertebra

Sacrum

Prolapsed intervertebral disc (viewed from above)

Lumbar spondylosis (viewed from the side)

Lower back problems can cause pinching of the nerves supplying the bladder as they exit the spinal canal, affecting bladder control.

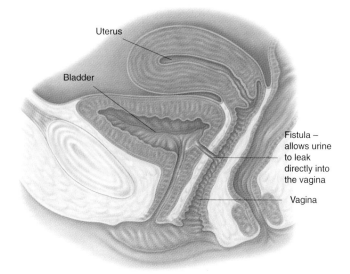

Fistula between the bladder and vagina.

cancer, because cancer and the radiotherapy weaken the muscles. They may also occur after an operation where the surfaces have become damaged, particularly after a hysterectomy. In other parts of the world the most common cause is abnormally long (obstructed) labour when giving birth. This leads to a pressure sore that erodes, usually between the bladder and the vagina. Fistulae may also be congenital, i.e. you may be born with them.

Fistulae are uncommon problems that require specialist care. They will sometimes heal without an operation, but this may take some weeks, during which time a catheter would be needed to keep the bladder empty. Operations for fistulae require great skill, and postoperative care, to help prevent a recurrence.

CONGENITAL DEFECTS

Congenital defects are conditions where a child is born with an alteration in the normal anatomy, such as an ectopic ureter. This is a condition where the ureter (the tube connecting the bladder with the kidney) does not connect with the bladder. Instead it is connected direct to the vagina, which again causes leaking as the bladder is bypassed. These are normally diagnosed in early life and treated appropriately.

KEY POINTS

✓ Other health problems can be linked with incontinence

✓ Surgery should aim to treat all problems at once

✓ Treatment needs to be tailored to individual needs

Managing the problem: aids and appliances

Over the last 20 years there has been an increase in the number of companies producing incontinence products as the true size of the problem has become apparent. The market for aids and appliances exists because most women prefer to deal with their incontinence themselves rather than seeking professional help.

WHAT DO YOU REQUIRE?

- What trouble does your incontinence cause?
- Do you leak small amounts often or large amounts infrequently?
- When does it trouble you? At night or only during exercise?
- How easy is it for you to change when you have leaked (does the pad have to act just as a stop-gap until you reach the toilet or is it going to have to protect you for several hours)?
- Do you need help to change or are you able to manage on your own?
- Can you easily remove a pad from a pouch within pants, or are nappies easier?
- How important is it to have a discreet small pad to allow tight-fitting clothes?
- Your size and shape may make different products more acceptable or more difficult for you to use

Unfortunately this can prove expensive and not always effective, as the appliances bought may be either unsuitable or incorrectly sized. They are available on the NHS and through the District Continence Advisory Service.

The aim of these products is to contain the problem sufficiently to allow 'social' continence. With this in mind there is a spectrum of products available from panty liners allowing simple discreet protection through to fail-safe absorbent pads similar to nappies, from underpads for seats and beds to catheters to keep the bladder permanently empty.

Most chemists now stock a wide selection of products. The key to success in the choice of product is assessment of your requirements.

The choice of incontinence aid is therefore based on many factors. Help is available through the Continence Foundation and the District Continence Advisory Service, who will advise you what can be done to limit the impact of your incontinence on your lifestyle and help you select the best appliance for your needs.

PANTY LINERS AND PADS

The simplest protection offered is panty liners, which can be discreet and unobtrusive but are very poor at absorbing urine. They are generally available everywhere and

CONSIDERATIONS IN CHOICE OF INCONTINENCE AID

- Size and shape
- Reliability
- Quantity of urine held
- Odour
- Concealability
- Comfort and skin irritability
- Price
- Accessibility/supply
- Disposable/reusable
- Ease of use/changing

are quite comfortable and easy to change. They offer only very limited protection and may require regular changing. Sometimes they can lead to problems as the plastic backing causes an increase in perspiration which can be mistaken for leakage. They are attractive because they are 'normal' for women to wear and hence not particularly associated with incontinence.

Pads with waterproof backing allow greater security. These are more absorbent than panty liners, but may still allow leakage around the edge of the pad. They also tend to be thicker, longer and wider. Some are shaped to allow a better fit. Heavier pads are available for severe leakage problems; for the best results these require stretch pants to hold them in position.

MARSUPIAL PANTS

Marsupial pants are waterproof pants with a separate changeable pad within a pocket. This allows the pad to be changed without needing to change the pants. Urine drains through the porous layer of the pants into the pad. The major advantage of this system is that it allows the pad to stay in place without repositioning. This is useful for someone with reduced dexterity who is likely to forget to reposition the pad after being in the toilet. The drawback is that the inner lining is not changed after incontinence and there is then one persistently dirty layer next to the skin.

There is now an increasing number of clothing companies marketing underwear with either waterproofed gussets or built-in pads. These products are helpful in improving body image and allow women to feel more normal in their choice of underwear.

NAPPIES

The most reliable of all systems, however, is an all-in-one pad, that is, disposable pants with built-in pads. Improvements in the design have resulted in better fit and therefore greater comfort; they are considerably lighter and better at containing leakage than older versions.

MATTRESS COVERS

There are a wide variety of covers available. The choice is dependent on the amount and frequency of leakage. A child who is occasionally wetting the bed, for example, will require a much lighter sheet than someone who empties their bladder every night and is likely to continue to do so. Newer designs of breathable fabrics tend to be more comfortable, but also more expensive.

UNDERPADS

There are a variety of underpads available that can be used for protection of furniture. The underpad works by collecting any leakage in a storage layer away from the skin. This protects the skin from sores caused by the irritation of long-term contact of the skin with urine.

KEY POINTS

✓ There is a range of products to help you manage incontinence

✓ Advice on products is available through the Continence Foundation and the District Continence Advisory Service

✓ The key to choosing the best product is an assessment of your requirements

What treatment is right for you?

If you have read this far, you will realise that incontinence is a complicated topic. There are many different types with many different causes. What they have in common is that treatment is available to relieve symptoms and improve the quality of your life. The big change that has happened in the past ten years is that tests are now available to identify precisely what is wrong. The treatment can then be tailored precisely to the cause.

The most common type of incontinence is stress incontinence which can almost always be controlled, and often completely cured by exercises or an operation. Surgery may not be possible in all cases because of poor general health, for example, but that does not mean that there is no treatment. There are well-tried alternatives, including drug treatments and a whole range of appliances.

The range of treatments is rapidly expanding as incontinence is increasingly seen as an important area of health care. This has resulted in an enormous improvement in treatment in recent years. No one is too old to be able to benefit. So ask for help: it is available through the NHS; your GP is your first port of call.

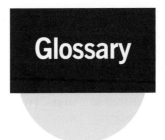

Glossary

cystitis This is commonly taken to mean pain on passing urine. It actually means an inflammation of the bladder. People usually refer to cystitis when they think they have an infection and mean frequency, urgency and dysuria.

detrusor muscle The muscle in the bladder wall which contracts during voiding.

dysuria Abnormal voiding, which may be painful or difficult.

enuresis Bedwetting, normally known as nocturnal enuresis, as it occurs at night.

frequency Having to pass urine more commonly than normal (normal is up to seven times a day) or more often than every two hours.

hesitancy A period of delay while waiting with the sensation of wanting to void before voiding begins.

micturition See voiding.

nocturia Having to get up at night, more than once, after falling asleep, to pass urine. This is unusual in a normal person under the age of around 60.

After this age it is normal to need to pass urine about once more for every decade over 60, i.e. a 70 year old would be expected to pass urine twice at night and an 80 year old three times.

perineum The area between the vagina and the anus.

prolapse The displacement of part of the body from its normal position. The term is usually used in association with changes of the pelvic organs 'prolapsing' into the vagina.

strangury The sensation of wanting to pass urine but being unable to do so.

stress incontinence The leakage of urine on raised intra-abdominal pressure (leakage with coughing, sneezing or exercise).

ultrasound A test used to look at the body using sound waves to build up a picture.

ureter The tube connecting the kidney to the bladder.

urethra The tube connecting the bladder to the outside.

urethral sphincter The bladder neck; the ring of muscles at the bottom of the bladder, which seals the bladder shut between voidings.

urge incontinence Urgency associated with leakage.

urgency The sudden and uncontrollable desire to pass urine.

urine Waste product of the body filtered by the kidneys.

urodynamic detrusor overactivity An unstable bladder.

voiding Emptying the bladder/ urination/passing urine/micturition.

Useful addresses

Association of Chartered Physiotherapists in Women's Health
c/o Chartered Society of Physiotherapists
14 Bedford Row
London WC1R 4ED
Tel: 020 7242 1941
Email: webmaster@womensphysio.com
Website: www.womensphysio.com

Continence Foundation
307 Hatton Square
16 Baldwins Gardens
London EC1N 7RJ
Helpline: 0805 345 0165 (Mon–Fri 9.00am–1.00pm)
Tel: 020 7404 6875
Fax: 020 7404 6876
Email:
continence.foundation@dial.pipex.com
Website: www.continence-foundation.org.uk

Provides information and advice on bladder and bowel problems and encourages people to seek the help on offer.

***In*contact**
United House
North Road
London N7 9DP
Tel: 0870 770 3246
Fax: 0870 770 3249
Email: info@incontact.org
Website: www.incontact.org

Offers information and support to people who have bladder and bowel conditions and to their carers. Publishes a quarterly newsletter.

Interstitial Cystitis Support Group
76 High Street
Stony Stratford
Bucks MK11 1AH
Tel/fax: 01908 569169
Email: info@interstitialcystitis.co.uk
Website: www.interstitialcystitis.co.uk

Gives support to people with interstitial cystitis, and their families and friends.

PromoCon
Redbank House, 4 St Chad's Street
Cheetham
Manchester M8 8QA
Tel: 0161 834 2001
Fax: 0161 214 5961
Email:
promocon2001@disabledliving.co.uk
Website: www.promocon2001.co.uk

THE INTERNET AS A SOURCE OF FURTHER INFORMATION

After reading this book, you may feel that you would like further information on the subject. One source is the internet and there are a great many websites with useful information about medical disorders, related charities and support groups. Some websites, however, have unhelpful and inaccurate information. Many are sponsored by commercial organisations or raise revenue by advertising, but nevertheless aim to provide impartial and trustworthy health information. Others may be reputable but you should be aware that they may be biased in their recommendations. Remember that treatment advertised on international websites may not be available in the UK.

Unless you know the address of the specific website that you want to visit (for example, familydoctor. co.uk), you may find the following guidelines helpful when searching the internet.

There are several different sorts of websites that you can use to look for information, the main ones being search engines, directories and portals.

Search engines and directories

There are many search engines and directories that all use different algorithms (procedures for computation) to return different results when you do a search. Search engines use computer programs called spiders, which crawl the web on a daily basis to search individual pages within a site and then queue them ready for listing in their database.

Directories, however, consider a site as a whole and use the description and information that was provided with the site when it was submitted to the directory to decide whether a site matches the searcher's needs. For both there is little or no selection in terms of quality of information, although engines and directories do try to impose rules about decency and content. Popular search engines in the UK include:

google.co.uk
aol.co.uk
msn.co.uk
lycos.co.uk
hotbot.co.uk
overture.com
ask.co.uk

espotting.com
looksmart.co.uk
alltheweb.com
uk.altavista.com

The two biggest directories are:

yahoo.com
dmoz.org

Portals
Portals are doorways to the internet that provide links to useful sites, news and other services, and may also provide search engine services (such as msn.co.uk). Many portals charge for putting their clients' sites high up in your list of search results. The quality of the websites listed depends on the selection criteria used in compiling the portal, although portals focused on a specific group, such as medical information portals, may have more rigorous inclusion criteria than other searchable websites. Examples of medical portals can be found at:

nhsdirect.nhs.uk
patient.co.uk

Links to many British medical charities will be found at the Association of Medical Research Charities (www.amrc.org.uk) and Charity Choice (www.charitychoice.co.uk).

Search phrases
Be specific when entering a search phrase. Searching for information on 'cancer' could give astrological information as well as medical: 'lung cancer' would be a better choice. Either use the engine's advanced search feature and ask for the exact phrase, or put the phrase in quotes – 'lung cancer' – as this will link the words. Adding 'uk' to your search phrase will bring up mainly British websites, so a good search would be 'lung cancer' uk (don't include uk within the quotes).

Always remember that the internet is international and unregulated. Although it holds a wealth of invaluable information, individual websites may be biased, out of date or just plain wrong. Family Doctor Publications accepts no responsibility for the content of links published in their series.

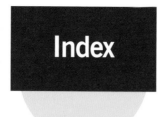

Index